Pregnancy Tips and Tricks from a Mom You Don't Know

Pregnancy Tips and Tricks from a Mom You Don't Know

This Mom's Insight on Pregnancy and Babies

Cathleen Holmes

ISBN 978-1-4583-5387-0

This book is dedicated to my husband and kids for giving me the world and E. Rapier, who inspired this idea.

Table of Contents

I realize that some of these topics are the subject of heated discussions between moms everywhere. However, in the spirit of motherhood and laughing at the things we just cannot control on the road we take to get there, I would like to pass along some of the things I've learned during *my* experiences on *my* roads that led us to three kids.

This book gives you the good, the bad, and the ugly. I hope to offend no one and to make many laugh. After all, if we couldn't laugh, what a *long* forty weeks it would be!

Pregnancy is a wonderfully crazy and joyfully terrifying ride for women and their husbands everywhere. It's unpredictable and hilarious, fun and embarrassing. It is literally the best of times and the worst of times all rolled into one.

Many a pregnancy tip, tale, or story has been told, but not many as honestly as what you will see here. I am a woman who loves being pregnant, but wears it like a sweaty, fat suit. The way I see it, why not pass along my small bit of mom wisdom and laugh at it all in the process?

In my opinion, this is the stuff that gets us through it all—still clinging to a shred of our womanly sanity. So put on your big-girl pants and read on. The conversation may not be pretty, but it sure is funny.

Tips and Tricks during Pregnancy:

1. I learned the hard way with my first baby that the most important thing is to keep your pregnant butt *moving!*—even if all you do is take a daily walk. I didn't with our first (who is now seven) and gained seventy pounds! Eeek!

   I have not been on a scale since, and that is no lie. This mom was scarred for life by the digital number glaring back at not just me, but the nurse weighing me for delivery prep. Not cool. Which leads me right into number two …

2. Other than brownies, pregnancy workout DVDs are every woman's best friend for ten months. (Yes, for those who don't yet know, they have extended pregnancy an entire month—used to be nine, now it's ten. Why not go for 11?)

Those DVDs are the number-one way to get your butt moving without people seeing you jiggle all over a gym, it's bad enough when we're alone! There is a mind-numbing array to choose from, meaning that *every* lady during any trimester can work those cheese doodles off! No excuses!

3.   A belly support belt will *save* your back! It seems like there is nothing worse than throwing out your back picking up a toddler or giant basket of clothes.

Try having it happen when you're just trying to haul your pregnant ass off of a friend's couch or, even worse, a chair in a *public place*. Humiliating!

Why take that chance? The minute you feel your lower back is officially compromised by the weight of your belly, slap one of those babies on and keep on truckin' toward your due date!

4.   It is *never* too soon to start stocking up on diapers. Seriously, once you've passed the point (you know you have one) where you no longer feel like you are jinxing the pregnancy, start stocking up!

Don't forget, you are going to need *all sizes* not just newborn! Don't just fill a closet with fifty packs of teeny-tiny diapers. You will be mad as heck when you have to try to find a way to get rid of a bunch of miniature diapers that cost good money once your baby is too big for them!

If you're a first-time mom and worried about buying a brand before you try it on your baby, just opt for the one your hospital uses. If it works there (and it will) it will work at home too! Really!

At the end of the day, a diaper is a diaper, people, and as long as your baby doesn't have a skin reaction, it's as good as every other diaper out there. Just buy what suits your budget, keep your eyes open for great deals, and stop listening to the mom next door!

5.   Never, ever forget the power of a good BJ for your husband when you couldn't care less about "putting out" for days, weeks, or months at a time. This one simple act will keep your husband happy, and he *will* help you out more.

I promise.

If you acknowledge his needs, you will actually have a shot in hell of him not only caring about yours, but caring even more than usual! You too can make the miracle of all miracles happen!

6.   A body pillow will change your pregnant night life! I love them all, no matter their shape or size. The simple fact of not having to haul a million pounds of stomach from side to side all night makes the investment worth it.

Your husband will probably hate any body pillow you bring home for obvious reasons. I've found the solution to this issue is, once again, a BJ as suggested in number five. It works like a charm every time, and a happy man is not a complaining man. He will suddenly cease to notice your beloved, temporary bed buddy.

7.   For the duration of ten months, your pantry should *always* contain an emergency stash of your favorite macaroni and cheese. There is something about this comfort food that satisfies pregnant women everywhere!

It can be made quickly at any time of day or night, making it easy to put away an entire box with your family being none the wiser. If no one saw the calories, they did not exist. It's true, I swear!

8.   Do *not* wait until your third trimester to start baby's nursery. If you do wait, please know that you risk finding yourself eight-and-a-half-months pregnant, standing on a chair at 11:00 p.m. trying to stamp a border around the darn ceiling of your new baby's room.

You will also probably find yourself buying *way* too many things you will never use in your last-minute frenzy to not be a "bad mom" who brings the baby home to a lacking nursery. When you only have two seconds to think, *everything* on the Newborn Must-Have list will seem like an actual must-have.

What's the bottom line? This is just not the time to let procrastination win. Get off your ass and start that nursery!

9. Until my third pregnancy, I had *no idea* that you could actually get your own baby doppler (a portable ultrasound). Not only can you get your own, you can also choose between buying *and* renting. Awesome!

   These are beyond handy for any pregnant mom who is nearing the end of the first trimester, especially after those extra-freaky baby dreams that plague us at one point or another. Baby dreams such as the multiples dream. Nooo! With a doppler, you can reassure your pounding heart within seconds that there is, indeed, still just one baby in there!

10. Lotion, lotion, lotion. I realize that many say stretch marks are hereditary. However, I truly believe that if you do not use lotion, you are guaranteed to look like a road map when it's all said and done. I have seen it with my own two eyes. The more I use, the fewer I seem to get. Don't buy into that "pregnancy lotion" crap either—all kinds work.

11. A bag of Pillsbury frozen biscuits and a jar of jam may *seem* like your best friend when you are nine months pregnant. In the end, they are not. Bake yourself one, maybe two, and move the hell on!

12. If you are planning to breast-feed, start pricing breast pumps *now*! They are expensive and a must-have if you plan on date nights, peeing alone when you have to, or doing any other general life activity when your baby needs your breast milk.

Never pass up a great deal on a new or used pump. Yes, I said it: *used.* They are easily sterilized and will save you a lot of money! Having your first baby (or even your fourth) does *not* mean you have to break the bank or go without!

13. Inevitably, at some point during your pregnancy, your husband will be picking up food for you.

Tacos, for example. Please, try to not just restrain yourself, but also hide your rage when he hands over, for example, a one-pound bean burrito with everything on it instead of the golden, wonderful, must-have-beef tacos that you were expecting.

Subdue the animal rage when he hands you a California Dreamin' (with limp, freaky bacon and baby-poop-looking avocado mush) sub sandwich, when all you asked for was turkey with lettuce, tomato, and mayo because—he was just trying to "spice things up" for you.

He knows not what he does. At the end of the day, it is simply your husband trying to say he loves you during this difficult time. After all, it is only because he cannot seem to understand the number-one rule of pregnancy: do *not* mess with a pregnant woman's food or food orders, subject to penalty by law!

Simply hide your anger and smile, have a small cry in private if it was a particularly important food item you just *had* to have, and move on. There is no other choice, and once you have your baby, you will again realize that your marriage really *is* more important to you than a Snickers bar.

14. Read, in order, *Belly Laughs* by Jenny McCarthy (hilarious, straightforward humor at a time when it is much needed!) and *What to Expect When You're Expecting,* the holy grail of pregnancy books. My ninety-two-year-old grandma declares it to be the best idea for women since the girdle— and, given the history of women, that's saying something!

Jenny loosens you up with a few good laughs and gross, giant belly tidbits before you dive right into the overwhelming reality of exactly what you are in for on this ride. If you're the hard-core type, feel free to reverse the order.

15.   Need a foolproof way to pull yourself out of a pregnancy slump? Pregnancy movies to the rescue!

There is something about seeing our own kind hauling their pregnant selves around cutely on screen that will make you feel like you're not alone.

You aren't the only whale! Someone else does understand exactly how stupid husbands can be! There are cravings weirder than yours!

Grab a couch, some ice cream, and a copy of *Nine Months* or *Look Who's Talking,* and I guarantee you'll be right as rain in no time and staring your next trimester boldly in the face without a flinch.

NOTES

NOTES

There is nothing put-together about a post-baby mama. Everything is gross and everywhere. You're tired and trying to find your dignity and some sense of body again.

For me, this time was plagued with nightmares about my insanely clear memory of the exact moment during delivery that, instead of pushing out a baby, I pushed out a huge fart—directly into my doctor's face.

That was a few minutes before I told him, point blank, that I was going to kill him. Oh, the absolute *horror!*

This is the very same doctor who I will have to face again in a mere six months for round three. A man will *never* fully understand what we go through for our family. Regardless of the shame and exhaustion, the bleary-eyed days march on.

Thankfully they march ever-closer to easier days that involve more uninterrupted sleep and, of course, the enjoyment of your ever-growing, sweet little baby.

Tips and Tricks: Post-Delivery:

1. I will start with the one I find most pertinent. You *can* and *should* bathe. Simply put, put the baby in a bouncer (another newborn must-have!) and bring it into the bathroom with you. Voilà! Shower time!

    I don't understand, nor do I trust, women who don't know this and just do not bathe. Something is wrong with that picture.

2. The Belly Bandit is the best thing *ever!* I discovered it while pregnant with baby number two, and I was cleared by my doctor to wear it as soon as the day I left the hospital.

    There is a whole connection I was unaware of with 'binding' your belly and it shrinking back to a (more) normal size more quickly than without it. It doesn't hurt or feel uncomfortable, and it creates the illusion of your tummy being *a lot* flatter than it is.

However, I do have one warning: it seems that the tighter you bind it, the louder the Velcro ripping sound is when you bend over. Awesome!

For that reason, I only wear mine at home, but that hasn't stopped it from working wonderfully for me!

3. *Spanx! Spanx! Spanx!* The miracle of all miracles, post-baby! There are a ton of undergarments that will fit under *any* type of clothing. They will give you a glorious glimpse of the you that you were and the you that you will be again!

4. If you breast-feed, you will want to buy stock in nipple cream. It is *that* great. It will be your saving grace in a sea of crazy nipple pain. It will be the calm to your nipple storm.

    To make the process even more painless, I put the cream directly on one of those disposable cotton breast pads, then put it between my bra and breast. No need to get your fingers gross and cause yourself more pain in the process!

    Reminder: Be sure to check yourself in a mirror before leaving the house. Nothing is a dead giveaway to boob problems like a wrinkled up or folded boob pad sitting awkwardly in a bra and showing right through your T-shirt. We all deserve our dignity, after all—breast-feeding or not. Lots of button-down shirts will make this entire process a hell of a lot easier on you.

5. Hemorrhoid medicated pads combined with hemorrhoid cream will make it possible to actually sit down or stand up without crying out after an ipisioto-whatchamacallit. It may even make it so you don't—*gasp!*—need a donut pillow for the next four weeks.

    If that isn't quite enough and you still feel like your lady junk may fall off, there is a special spray that the doctor can get you (though they never seem to mention this product upfront). That spray is guaranteed to bring enough relief to unpinch your face for a few hours.

6.   If it's an option for you, one of the prepared meal plans like Weight Watchers is *great* for a new mom trying to drop some pounds. I see results quickly—and the best part is that you are back to making one meal at a time for the rest of your family, since yours is already made. Fabulous!

7.   Read, in order, *Baby Laughs* by Jenny McCarthy (even more hilarious!) and then *What to Expect the First Year*. Once again, Jenny eases you into the overwhelming look at what you are in for the first 365 days of this new little person's life.

8.   Whether or not you are breast-feeding, a bottle warmer in your baby's room is a midnight lifesaver! We set up a little bottle station on the dresser with formula or pumped breast milk and pre-measured water to put in the warmer. This way, you are able to stumble in half awake and whip up a quick bottle without having to actually wake up and think at 2:38 a.m. (much less go to the kitchen). Your tired eyes will thank you after a few nights of easier feedings.

9.   This next one is going to rub a few moms the wrong way so, again, I will say I am not here to offend. All of us are not going to agree on everything.

      I have found that, when you're at home and you need a few minutes hands free (for various tasks or reasons), a *Baby Einstein* DVD will keep even an eight-week-old baby occupied long enough for you to finish that call with your sister, write an e-mail using two hands, or, heaven forbid, use the powder room for longer than thirty seconds. I see nothing wrong with this at all.

      Sometimes a mom needs two seconds to herself, or she will just lose her mind. Why the heck shouldn't she get those two seconds?

      Rest assured, I have noticed that, as far as my children go, A, who has seen said movies, is definitely just as smart as E, who was born before baby DVDs were a thing. A's brain has not been deformed or stunted from seeing a strawberry on a screen playing pleasant classical music for a few minutes at a time here and there. I am positive she will still succeed in life, just like her sister.

10. Post-delivery, the nurses will offer to take your baby for small periods of time so you can sleep. *Let them!* You will get much-needed blocks of uninterrupted sleep after the biggest ordeal your body could have ever imagined.

Trust me when I say, you *need* the sleep. I am not saying you should interfere with bonding or time with your baby. That would be silly. But when night falls and the nurse pops her head in, ignore that pulling ache, give yourself a brief chance for recovery, and nod for her to come on in. She will *not* steal your baby, and you'll be a better, more-rested mom in the end!

The flip side, as I learned the hard way—*twice*—is that you go home a sleep-deprived, exhausted, irrational, psycho lunatic who now feels overwhelmed as well. *Not good.* I will, in fact, be taking this wonderful advice myself this time around.

NOTES

NOTES

It bothers the hell out of me that moms withhold information from each other. In my world, withholding equals dishonesty, and what kind of friend are you if you can't be honest? We pride ourselves on being the communicating sex, so dammit, ladies, pour a glass of wine, rip the tape off your mouth, and talk about the unspoken!

Things Other Moms Don't Tell You:

1. Let's begin with the one with which I have the biggest bone to pick.

   The truth about childbirth. I am about to say the forbidden words, ladies. The one thing that we are, for whatever insane reason, not supposed to say to anyone, much less a soon-to-be, first-time mom.

   Childbirth is *scary as hell.* So, for Pete's sake, make sure you like your doctor! Allow me to clarify some. *Labor* is not scary as hell. *Childbirth* is scary as hell. The moment you hear the word *crowning* thrown out into the room and you know that baby is about to come out—that's scary as hell for a woman.

   Moms everywhere are yelling "fear monger!" at this book this very moment. Some women think that uttering those words is the worst, most hateful thing a veteran mom could say. I will never, ever understand that. There is no way I believe that every single woman isn't scared shitless when the time for delivery comes.

   In what reality is realizing you are going to push a *human* from your vagina not scary as hell? If this reality does indeed exist, please take me there, because it is in this reality that I would like to dwell with my loved ones.

   I don't care if this is your first baby or you are the Duggars, pushing a baby out is scary as hell. Even a birth that goes perfectly from start to finish, as deemed by the world of medicine, is scary as hell for the woman and probably the husband as well. How could it possibly not be?

Every player in the room knows exactly what this team is here for, and it isn't a touchdown, people. It's bloody, intense, horrifying, and awesome childbirth. To not only say it out loud, but to say it to *other women,* makes it possible for the rest of ladykind to actually prepare for what's coming. It gives a mom the chance to figure out her biggest fear(s) about the situation and find actual ways to understand or cope with them before the delivery instead of at the height of the chaos.

I mean, come on, I can't be the only one who sees talking about it as a positive.

2.   Watch out for the type of mom who will be the first to jump all over me for the what I stated in item number one, yet will not hesitate for one second to tell you that your baby must have some kind of developmental problem if he or she isn't already walking by the age *her* child was. I have talked to more than one poor friend after such a conversation, and it is not pretty! If you meet this woman, run the other way as fast as you can!

3.   You do, in fact, remember childbirth after the fact. There is no delivery amnesia. Even my doctor (a man) has tried to convince me of this forgetful condition. It is not true. You will in fact remember most of the ordeal.

However, it is true that the gift of your baby outweighs the craziness. I believe that it is the actual reason women do it over and over again. Not because the magical Forget-Everything Fairy paid her a visit while she slept in the hospital bed.

In my opinion, declaring it an event comparable to say, a horrific car accident, by stating that you have no memory of said events at all, makes childbirth sound a hell of a lot scarier than saying, "Yeah, having my baby was crazy, and it totally freaked me out!"

4. Unless you are a rare, elusive breed of female, (e.g., Nicole Kidman) you can and will still look seven months pregnant when you leave the hospital. This is a heartbreaking, real, and all-together shocking fact that most first-time moms are not aware of, and moms a few times over will never get used to.

    Pack your pregnancy clothes in that hospital bag, honey, because there won't be any miracles happening in that birthing suite other than the emerging life of your new baby, just come out of the womb. The buck stops there. Cry about it; then get used to it. It's only temporary, after all.

    One look at your baby, and things will seem brighter, even if you're still looking at the baby while wearing your maternity jeans!

5. Another hot button subject: drugs. To have the drugs or not to have the drugs, that is the question.

    I had an epidural with my first baby, and I always wondered if it was the right thing to do. I chose, once again, to have an epidural with the second baby. I don't know how long after it was administered that the problem happened, all I know is that I was suddenly in more pain than I had ever known.

    I couldn't even make words come out of my mouth around the pain to tell my husband something was wrong. Something was wrong all right; there was a kink in my damn drugs line! I was feeling full-on labor on my entire right side, but nothing at all on my left. I wouldn't wish that kind of pain on the devil.

    My anesthesiologist raced back to the hospital amidst a snowstorm to help my poor, laboring ass out. I found out in a brief, horrifying period of time that, without a doubt, having a baby is just not the time for *me* to Just Say No. Long live the epidural!

6.   If you don't plan on cosleeping, get your baby in the crib by the third or fourth week! They can and will sleep in their own room. You will regain a small piece of sanity that will help you get through the next few months. And your husband will have hope for a revived sex life one day in the near future.

7.   You will sound like an obese person who must be cut from his or her home the first time you work out after having a baby, no matter what. Do not be frightened. Accept it and soldier on, knowing that you are not the only one! We are all huffing and puffing right behind you, cursing those Fritos and that Boston cream pie.

8.   It seriously takes a year to get rid of all of that baby weight, so don't stress it. Unless you are one of the moms who has four to six hours per day to devote to working out, give yourself a freaking break and hang in there. Your favorite jeans *will* fit again one day! Make good food choices and get to huffing and puffing, and it *will* happen!

9.   If you need coffee to stay in the game, especially in the first few weeks or months, drink it! As long as you aren't acting like a caffeine junkie, you will not make your baby hyper by breastfeeding. You will not harm your baby by breastfeeding. Instead, you will be awake and alert enough to not be one of those moms who falls asleep in the shower or forgets her baby at the grocery store because she thinks her personal caffeine intake will alter her child for life.

10.   When it comes to a first baby, during the first few weeks you will probably be scared shitless that something you do will harm or kill your baby—that you will somehow twist off an arm during a changing or drop the baby on its head. All perfectly normal fears.

      You are going to be fine, and so is your baby. It's not just you. We all walk around worrying that we are potential baby killers when see how helpless the babies look in the beginning.

11. Other than the loss of your lovely sleep, newborn babies are actually *really easy* to take care of. Seriously. Yes, they cry. Yes, they poop. But that really is the worst of it.

Once you find your groove with your husband and your baby, things float along (generally) nicely in a sleep-deprived fog for those first few weeks. As the days drift on, your baby will nail down an internal schedule, and you'll stop worrying that he or she will break quite so easily.

In my opinion, the newborn stage is the only time your child will be easy. Instead of wasting that time complaining that you need more sleep, live it up, woman! This is by far easy street on the long child-rearing journey ahead.

My days on the journey to motherhood are almost over, but I happily find myself smack in the middle of actually *being* a mom. It's one giant whirlwind of wonderful and terrifying, easy and hard, all wrapped up in toys and pee pants. It's the greatest time I've ever had. One day, I will look back fondly with a tear in my eye at a small baby shoe or favorite blankie kept for its memories as I sit and remember the past. For now, I'm trying to be present in every single second of this poop-filled glory. I hope your journey is as fun-filled as mine—and never forget: we're all here, right behind you, with that same dazed look in our eyes!

NOTES

NOTES

Baby To Do List

1st Trimester To Do List

1.

2.

3.

4.

5.

6.

7.

8.

9.

10.

2nd Trimester To Do List

1.

2.

3.

4.

5.

6.

7.

8.

9.

10.

3rd Trimester To Do List

1.

2.

3.

4.

5.

6.

7.

8.

9.

10.

I firmly believe in making life with a newborn as easy as possible on mom and dad. Deciding what you do and don't need for yourself and your new baby can be stressful on both your nerves *and* your wallet. In my opinion, a mom doesn't need very many things to make the first few months go smoothly while everyone is adjusting. I also think it's possible to prepare for a baby without breaking the bank. The following are the things I just can't live without when I bring home a new baby.

For baby's room:

1. Crib/crib sheets
2. Bassinet
3. Bottle warmer
4. Swaddling blanket
5. Glider/Rocking chair
6. Onsies
7. Pants
8. Sleepers
9. Sound machine
10. Baby monitor
11. Changing table
12. Diapers/wipes
13. Arm & Hammer disposable diaper bags (so much better than a diaper pail!)

For your home:

1. Bottle scrubber
2. All-In-One Stroller/Car Seat System
3. Bottles (Even when breast feeding if you plan to pump!)
4. Bouncer
5. Baby swing
6. Changing pad
7. Arm & Hammer disposable diaper bags (so much better than a diaper pail!)
8. Spit-up cloths

For your car:

1. Baby view mirror
2. Spare diapers/wipes
3. At least one clean bottle
4. Spare spit-up cloth
5. Portable breast pump (If breast feeding)
6. Changing pad
7. Arm & Hammer disposable diaper bags (so much better than a diaper pail!)
8. Soothing music
9. Blanket
10. All-In-One Stroller/Car Seat System
11. Baby sling (Sometimes a stroller is just too much!)

To Buy

Mom's Resource Reminder

1.   Work-out DVD's
2.   Belly support belt
3.   Body pillow
4.   What To Expect When You're Expecting by: Heidi Murkoff
5.   Belly Laughs by: Jenny McCarthy
6.   Baby Doppler
7.   Nipple cream
8.   Breast pump
9.   Bouncer for baby
10. Bottle warmer
11. Baby Einstein DVD's
12. Spanx
13. Belly Bandit
14. Baby Laughs by: Jenny McCarthy
15. What To Expect The First Year by: Heidi Murkoff

To Buy

My Pregnancy Journal

Conception Date:

Due Date:

Date I found out I was pregnant:

1st Doctor's Appointment:

1st Ultrasound:

Cravings:

1st time I felt baby move:

Sex of Baby:

Date of my Baby Shower:

When/where I went into labor:

How I decorated baby's nursery:

1st Ultrasound Photo:

When:

Where:

How I felt:

My Pregnancy Journal
1st Trimester

My Pregnancy Journal
2nd Trimester

My Pregnancy Journal
3rd Trimester

About the Author

Cathleen Holmes is a stay-at-home mom of three fabulous kids and a wonderful husband in Estes Park, Colorado.

www.ingramcontent.com/pod-product-compliance
Lightning Source LLC
Chambersburg PA
CBHW050347290526
45785CB00006B/2672